HIGH FIBER FOODS LIST

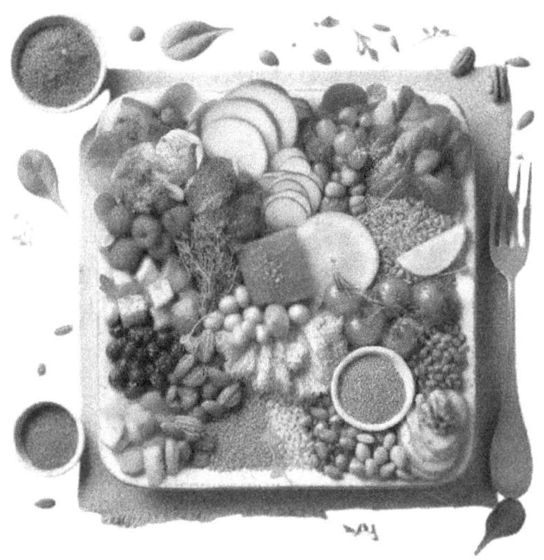

The comprehensive list on what to eat on high fiber diet

Tina Feldman

HIGH FIBER FOODS LIST

Table of Contents

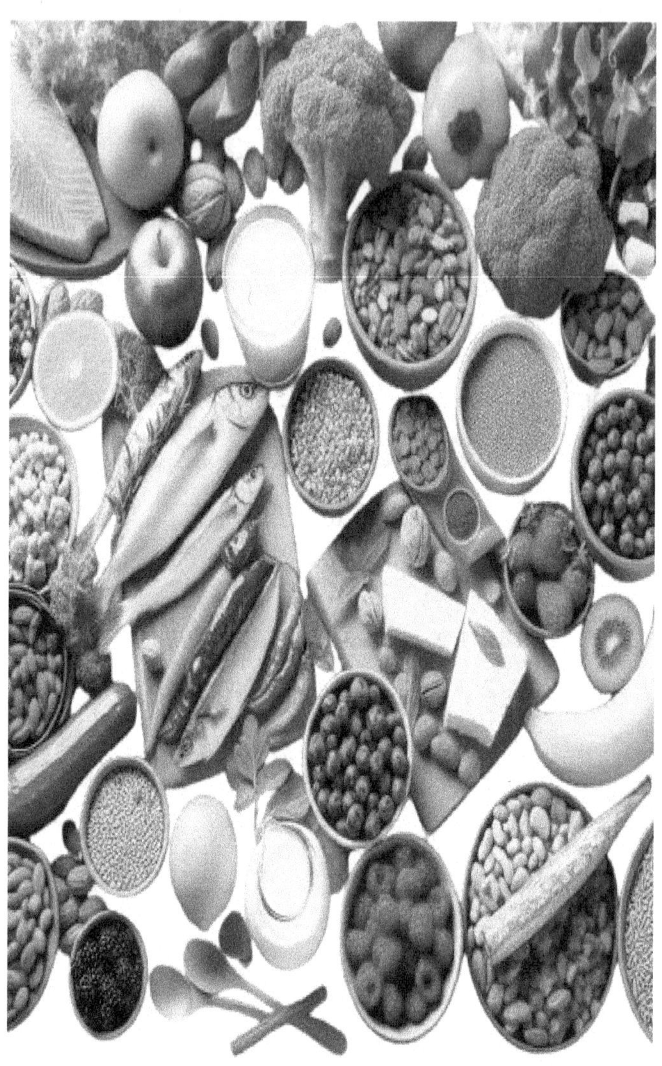

HIGH FIBER FOODS LIST

Introduction

Including high fiber foods into your diet is essential for promoting digestive health, maintaining a healthy weight, and reducing the risk of chronic diseases such as heart disease, diabetes, and certain types of cancer. Fiber, a type of carbohydrate found in plant-based foods, is known for its ability to aid digestion, regulate bowel movements, and promote feelings of fullness and satiety. Additionally, fiber plays a crucial role in supporting overall gut health by nourishing beneficial gut bacteria.

High fiber foods are typically whole, minimally processed foods that contain significant amounts of dietary fiber per serving. These foods include fruits, vegetables, legumes, whole grains, nuts, seeds. Incorporating a variety of high fiber foods into your meals and snacks can help you meet your daily fiber needs and enjoy a wide range of nutritional benefits.

In this list, we'll explore a diverse selection of high fiber foods, providing information on recommended daily fiber intake for different age groups and genders, fiber contents per serving, and other nutritional details. Whether you're looking to improve digestive health, manage your weight, or simply enjoy a balanced and nutritious diet, incorporating high fiber foods into your meals can be a delicious and satisfying way to support your overall well-being.

High fiber meal planning is essential for maintaining a healthy diet and promoting overall well-being. Incorporating ample amounts of fiber into your meals can help improve digestion, regulate blood sugar levels, lower cholesterol, and promote a healthy weight. Here are some detailed tips for high fiber meal planning:

Include a Variety of High Fiber Foods: Incorporate a diverse range of high fiber foods into your meals, including fruits, vegetables, whole grains, legumes, nuts, and seeds. Aim to include at least one high fiber food in each meal.

Choose Whole Grains: Opt for whole grains such as brown rice, quinoa, barley, oats, whole wheat bread, and whole grain pasta instead of refined grains. Whole grains contain more fiber, vitamins, minerals, and antioxidants compared to their refined counterparts.

Start with Breakfast: Begin your day with a high fiber breakfast to kickstart your metabolism and provide sustained energy throughout the morning. Choose fiber-rich options like oatmeal topped with fruits, whole grain toast with avocado, or a smoothie made with leafy greens and chia seeds.

Load Up on Fruits and Vegetables: Aim to fill half of your plate with fruits and vegetables at each meal. These colorful foods are naturally high in fiber, vitamins, minerals, and antioxidants. Incorporate a variety of fresh, frozen, or canned options to ensure you get a range of nutrients.

Snack Smart: Choose high fiber snacks to keep you satisfied between meals and prevent unhealthy cravings. Opt for options like raw vegetables with hummus, mixed nuts and seeds, whole fruit, Greek yogurt with berries, or whole grain crackers with nut butter.

Add Legumes to Meals: Incorporate beans, lentils, chickpeas, and other legumes into your meals to boost fiber content. They are versatile ingredients that can be added to soups, salads, stir-fries, wraps, and grain bowls.

Include Nuts and Seeds: Add nuts and seeds such as almonds, walnuts, chia seeds, and flaxseeds to your meals for extra fiber, healthy fats, and protein. Sprinkle them on top of yogurt, oatmeal, salads, or incorporate them into homemade granola or energy bars.

Read Food Labels: When grocery shopping, read food labels to identify high fiber options. Look for products that contain whole grains, fruits, vegetables, nuts, and seeds listed as the first few ingredients. Aim for foods with at least 3-5 grams of fiber per serving.

Cook at Home: Prepare meals at home whenever possible, as it allows you to control the ingredients and portion sizes. Experiment with different cooking methods such as steaming, roasting, sautéing, and grilling to enhance the flavor and texture of high fiber foods.

Stay Hydrated: Drink plenty of water throughout the day to help fiber move through your digestive system smoothly. Fiber absorbs water and swells in the digestive tract, so adequate hydration is essential for optimal digestion and bowel regularity.

Gradually Increase Fiber Intake: If you're not used to consuming a high fiber diet, gradually increase your fiber intake over time to allow your digestive system to adjust. Suddenly increasing fiber intake can cause digestive discomfort such as bloating and gas.

Consider Supplements: If you struggle to meet your daily fiber needs through food alone, consider incorporating a fiber supplement into your routine. However, it's essential to consult with a healthcare professional before starting any new supplement regimen.

High fiber foods list

Fruits

Raspberries:
Recommended Daily Intake:
Men: 38 grams
Women: 25 grams
Adult: 25-38 grams
Young (12-18 years): 25-31 grams
Kids (4-8 years): 25 grams
Fiber Content: Approximately 8 grams per cup (123 grams)
Other Nutrition Information: High in vitamin C, manganese, and antioxidants.

Blackberries:
Recommended Daily Intake:
Men: 38 grams
Women: 25 grams
Adult: 25-38 grams
Young (12-18 years): 25-31 grams
Kids (4-8 years): 25 grams
Fiber Content: Around 8 grams per cup (144 grams)
Other Nutrition Information: Rich in vitamin C, vitamin K, and manganese.

Avocado:

Recommended Daily Intake:
Men: 38 grams
Women: 25 grams
Adult: 25-38 grams
Young (12-18 years): 25-31 grams
Kids (4-8 years): 25 grams
Fiber Content: Roughly 10 grams per medium-sized avocado
Other Nutrition Information: High in healthy fats, potassium, vitamin K, and folate.

Guava:
Recommended Daily Intake:
Men: 38 grams
Women: 25 grams
Adult: 25-38 grams
Young (12-18 years): 25-31 grams
Kids (4-8 years): 25 grams
Fiber Content: Approximately 9 grams per cup (165 grams)
Other Nutrition Information: Rich in vitamin C, vitamin A, and antioxidants.

Pear:
Recommended Daily Intake:
Men: 38 grams
Women: 25 grams
Adult: 25-38 grams
Young (12-18 years): 25-31 grams
Kids (4-8 years): 25 grams
Fiber Content: About 6 grams per medium-sized pear
Other Nutrition Information: Good source of vitamin C, potassium, and antioxidants.

Apple (with skin):
Recommended Daily Intake:
Men: 38 grams
Women: 25 grams
Adult: 25-38 grams
Young (12-18 years): 25-31 grams
Kids (4-8 years): 25 grams
Fiber Content: Around 4 grams per medium-sized apple
Other Nutrition Information: Contains vitamin C, potassium, and various antioxidants.

Prunes (Dried Plums):
Recommended Daily Intake:
Men: 38 grams
Women: 25 grams
Adult: 25-38 grams
Young (12-18 years): 25-31 grams
Kids (4-8 years): 25 grams
Fiber Content: Roughly 12 grams per half cup (85 grams)
Other Nutrition Information: High in vitamin K, potassium, and antioxidants.

Kiwi:
Recommended Daily Intake:
Men: 38 grams
Women: 25 grams
Adult: 25-38 grams

Young (12-18 years): 25-31 grams
Kids (4-8 years): 25 grams
Fiber Content: Approximately 5 grams per medium-sized kiwi
Other Nutrition Information: Rich in vitamin C, vitamin K, and antioxidants.

Oranges:
Recommended Daily Intake:
Men: 38 grams
Women: 25 grams
Adult: 25-38 grams
Young (12-18 years): 25-31 grams
Kids (4-8 years): 25 grams
Fiber Content: Around 3 grams per medium-sized orange
Other Nutrition Information: High in vitamin C, potassium, and antioxidants.

Figs:
Recommended Daily Intake:
Men: 38 grams
Women: 25 grams
Adult: 25-38 grams
Young (12-18 years): 25-31 grams
Kids (4-8 years): 25 grams
Fiber Content: Roughly 7 grams per 3 dried figs
Other Nutrition Information: Good source of potassium, calcium, and antioxidants.

Legumes and Beans

Lentils:
Recommended Daily Intake:
Men: 38 grams
Women: 25 grams
Adult: 25-38 grams
Young (12-18 years): 25-31 grams
Kids (4-8 years): 14 grams
Fiber Content: Approximately 15.6 grams per cup (cooked)
Other Nutrition Information: High in protein, iron, folate, and potassium.

Black Beans:
Recommended Daily Intake:
Men: 38 grams
Women: 25 grams
Adult: 25-38 grams
Young (12-18 years): 25-31 grams
Kids (4-8 years): 14 grams
Fiber Content: Roughly 15 grams per cup (cooked)
Other Nutrition Information: Rich in protein, iron, magnesium, and antioxidants.

Chickpeas (Garbanzo Beans):
Recommended Daily Intake:
Men: 38 grams

Women: 25 grams
Adult: 25-38 grams
Young (12-18 years): 25-31 grams
Kids (4-8 years): 14 grams
Fiber Content: Around 12.5 grams per cup (cooked)
Other Nutrition Information: High in protein, folate, manganese, and phosphorus.

Split Peas:
Recommended Daily Intake:
Men: 38 grams
Women: 25 grams
Adult: 25-38 grams
Young (12-18 years): 25-31 grams
Kids (4-8 years): 14 grams
Fiber Content: Approximately 16.3 grams per cup (cooked)
Other Nutrition Information: Good source of protein, vitamin B1, and potassium.

Kidney Beans:
Recommended Daily Intake:
Men: 38 grams
Women: 25 grams
Adult: 25-38 grams
Young (12-18 years): 25-31 grams
Kids (4-8 years): 14 grams
Fiber Content: Roughly 13.1 grams per cup (cooked)
Other Nutrition Information: High in protein, iron, potassium, and antioxidants.

Pinto Beans:
Recommended Daily Intake:

Men: 38 grams
Women: 25 grams
Adult: 25-38 grams
Young (12-18 years): 25-31 grams
Kids (4-8 years): 14 grams
Fiber Content: Around 15.4 grams per cup (cooked)
Other Nutrition Information: Rich in protein, folate, magnesium, and manganese.

Black-eyed Peas:
Recommended Daily Intake:
Men: 38 grams
Women: 25 grams
Adult: 25-38 grams
Young (12-18 years): 25-31 grams
Kids (4-8 years): 14 grams
Fiber Content: Approximately 11.2 grams per cup (cooked)
Other Nutrition Information: High in protein, folate, iron, and potassium.

Adzuki Beans:
Recommended Daily Intake:
Men: 38 grams
Women: 25 grams
Adult: 25-38 grams
Young (12-18 years): 25-31 grams
Kids (4-8 years): 14 grams
Fiber Content: Roughly 17.3 grams per cup (cooked)
Other Nutrition Information: Good source of protein, folate, and potassium.

Soybeans:

Recommended Daily Intake:
Men: 38 grams
Women: 25 grams
Adult: 25-38 grams
Young (12-18 years): 25-31 grams
Kids (4-8 years): 14 grams
Fiber Content: Around 8.6 grams per half cup (cooked)
Other Nutrition Information: High in protein, iron, calcium, and healthy fats.

Lima Beans:
Recommended Daily Intake:
Men: 38 grams
Women: 25 grams
Adult: 25-38 grams
Young (12-18 years): 25-31 grams
Kids (4-8 years): 14 grams
Fiber Content: Approximately 13.2 grams per cup (cooked)
Other Nutrition Information: Rich in protein, iron, potassium, and folate.

Vegetables

Broccoli:
Recommended Daily Intake:
Men: 38 grams
Women: 25 grams
Adult: 25-38 grams
Young (12-18 years): 25-31 grams
Kids (4-8 years): 14 grams

Fiber Content: Approximately 5.1 grams per cup (91 grams) of chopped broccoli
Other Nutrition Information: High in vitamin C, vitamin K, folate, and antioxidants.

Brussels Sprouts:
Recommended Daily Intake:
Men: 38 grams
Women: 25 grams
Adult: 25-38 grams
Young (12-18 years): 25-31 grams
Kids (4-8 years): 14 grams
Fiber Content: Roughly 4.1 grams per cup (88 grams) of cooked Brussels sprouts
Other Nutrition Information: Rich in vitamin K, vitamin C, folate, and antioxidants.

Artichokes:
Recommended Daily Intake:
Men: 38 grams
Women: 25 grams
Adult: 25-38 grams
Young (12-18 years): 25-31 grams
Kids (4-8 years): 14 grams
Fiber Content: Approximately 10.3 grams per medium-sized artichoke
Other Nutrition Information: High in antioxidants, vitamin C, vitamin K, and magnesium.

Spinach:
Recommended Daily Intake:
Men: 38 grams
Women: 25 grams

Adult: 25-38 grams
Young (12-18 years): 25-31 grams
Kids (4-8 years): 14 grams
Fiber Content: Around 2.4 grams per cup (cooked)
Other Nutrition Information: Rich in iron, vitamin K, vitamin A, and antioxidants.

Kale:
Recommended Daily Intake:
Men: 38 grams
Women: 25 grams
Adult: 25-38 grams
Young (12-18 years): 25-31 grams
Kids (4-8 years): 14 grams
Fiber Content: Approximately 2.6 grams per cup (chopped)
Other Nutrition Information: High in vitamin K, vitamin A, vitamin C, and antioxidants.

Sweet Potatoes:
Recommended Daily Intake:
Men: 38 grams
Women: 25 grams
Adult: 25-38 grams
Young (12-18 years): 25-31 grams
Kids (4-8 years): 14 grams
Fiber Content: Roughly 4 grams per medium-sized sweet potato (with skin)
Other Nutrition Information: Rich in vitamin A, vitamin C, potassium, and antioxidants.

Carrots:
Recommended Daily Intake:

Men: 38 grams
Women: 25 grams
Adult: 25-38 grams
Young (12-18 years): 25-31 grams
Kids (4-8 years): 14 grams
Fiber Content: Around 3.6 grams per cup (chopped)
Other Nutrition Information: High in vitamin A, vitamin K, vitamin C, and antioxidants.

Peas:
Recommended Daily Intake:
Men: 38 grams
Women: 25 grams
Adult: 25-38 grams
Young (12-18 years): 25-31 grams
Kids (4-8 years): 14 grams
Fiber Content: Approximately 8.8 grams per cup (cooked)
Other Nutrition Information: Rich in protein, vitamin K, vitamin C, and folate.

Cauliflower:
Recommended Daily Intake:
Men: 38 grams
Women: 25 grams
Adult: 25-38 grams
Young (12-18 years): 25-31 grams
Kids (4-8 years): 14 grams
Fiber Content: Roughly 2.5 grams per cup (chopped)
Other Nutrition Information: High in vitamin C, vitamin K, folate, and antioxidants.

Green Beans:

Recommended Daily Intake:
Men: 38 grams
Women: 25 grams
Adult: 25-38 grams
Young (12-18 years): 25-31 grams
Kids (4-8 years): 14 grams
Fiber Content: Approximately 4 grams per cup (cooked)
Other Nutrition Information: Good source of vitamin C, vitamin K, and folate.

Nuts and Seeds

Almonds:
Recommended Daily Intake:
Men: 38 grams
Women: 25 grams
Adult: 25-38 grams
Young (12-18 years): 20-31 grams
Kids (4-8 years): 14 grams
Fiber Content: Approximately 3.5 grams per ounce (28 grams)
Other Nutrition Information: Rich in vitamin E, magnesium, and healthy fats.

Chia Seeds:
Recommended Daily Intake:
Men: 38 grams
Women: 25 grams
Adult: 25-38 grams
Young (12-18 years): 20-31 grams
Kids (4-8 years): 14 grams

Fiber Content: Around 10 grams per ounce (28 grams)
Other Nutrition Information: High in omega-3 fatty acids, calcium, and antioxidants.
Flaxseeds:
Recommended Daily Intake:
Men: 38 grams
Women: 25 grams
Adult: 25-38 grams
Young (12-18 years): 20-31 grams
Kids (4-8 years): 14 grams
Fiber Content: Approximately 8 grams per ounce (28 grams)
Other Nutrition Information: Good source of omega-3 fatty acids, lignans, and protein.

Pumpkin Seeds (Pepitas):
Recommended Daily Intake:
Men: 38 grams
Women: 25 grams
Adult: 25-38 grams
Young (12-18 years): 20-31 grams
Kids (4-8 years): 14 grams
Fiber Content: Roughly 5 grams per ounce (28 grams)
Other Nutrition Information: High in iron, magnesium, zinc, and antioxidants.

Sunflower Seeds:
Recommended Daily Intake:
Men: 38 grams
Women: 25 grams
Adult: 25-38 grams

Young (12-18 years): 20-31 grams
Kids (4-8 years): 14 grams
Fiber Content: Around 3.6 grams per ounce (28 grams)
Other Nutrition Information: Rich in vitamin E, selenium, and healthy fats.

Walnuts:
Recommended Daily Intake:
Men: 38 grams
Women: 25 grams
Adult: 25-38 grams
Young (12-18 years): 20-31 grams
Kids (4-8 years): 14 grams
Fiber Content: Approximately 2 grams per ounce (28 grams)
Other Nutrition Information: High in omega-3 fatty acids, antioxidants, and protein.

Hazelnuts (Filberts):
Recommended Daily Intake:
Men: 38 grams
Women: 25 grams
Adult: 25-38 grams
Young (12-18 years): 20-31 grams
Kids (4-8 years): 14 grams
Fiber Content: Roughly 2.7 grams per ounce (28 grams)
Other Nutrition Information: Good source of vitamin E, magnesium, and healthy fats.

Pistachios:
Recommended Daily Intake:

Men: 38 grams
Women: 25 grams
Adult: 25-38 grams
Young (12-18 years): 20-31 grams
Kids (4-8 years): 14 grams
Fiber Content: Around 3 grams per ounce (28 grams)
Other Nutrition Information: High in protein, potassium, and antioxidants.

Sesame Seeds:
Recommended Daily Intake:
Men: 38 grams
Women: 25 grams
Adult: 25-38 grams
Young (12-18 years): 20-31 grams
Kids (4-8 years): 14 grams
Fiber Content: Approximately 3.5 grams per ounce (28 grams)
Other Nutrition Information: Rich in calcium, iron, and antioxidants.

Peanuts:
Recommended Daily Intake:
Men: 38 grams
Women: 25 grams
Adult: 25-38 grams
Young (12-18 years): 20-31 grams
Kids (4-8 years): 14 grams
Fiber Content: Roughly 2.5 grams per ounce (28 grams)
Other Nutrition Information: High in protein, monounsaturated fats, and various vitamins and minerals.

Quinoa:
Recommended Daily Intake:
Men: 38 grams
Women: 25 grams
Adult: 25-38 grams
Young (12-18 years): 20-31 grams
Kids (4-8 years): 14 grams
Fiber Content: Approximately 5 grams per cooked cup (185 grams)
Other Nutrition Information: High in protein, contains all essential amino acids, rich in magnesium, iron, and antioxidants.

Oats:
Recommended Daily Intake:
Men: 38 grams
Women: 25 grams
Adult: 25-38 grams
Young (12-18 years): 20-31 grams
Kids (4-8 years): 14 grams
Fiber Content: Around 4 grams per cooked cup (234 grams)
Other Nutrition Information: Source of beta-glucan, a soluble fiber, which helps lower cholesterol levels. Rich in manganese, phosphorus, and antioxidants.

Barley:
Recommended Daily Intake:
Men: 38 grams
Women: 25 grams
Adult: 25-38 grams
Young (12-18 years): 20-31 grams
Kids (4-8 years): 14 grams
Fiber Content: Approximately 6 grams per cooked cup (157 grams)
Other Nutrition Information: Contains beta-glucan and insoluble fiber, which promote gut health. Good source of manganese, selenium, and vitamin B6.

Brown Rice:
Recommended Daily Intake:
Men: 38 grams
Women: 25 grams
Adult: 25-38 grams
Young (12-18 years): 20-31 grams
Kids (4-8 years): 14 grams
Fiber Content: Roughly 4 grams per cooked cup (195 grams)
Other Nutrition Information: Contains resistant starch, which acts as a prebiotic and supports healthy digestion. Rich in selenium, magnesium, and antioxidants.

Bulgur Wheat:
Recommended Daily Intake:
Men: 38 grams
Women: 25 grams
Adult: 25-38 grams
Young (12-18 years): 20-31 grams

Kids (4-8 years): 14 grams
Fiber Content: Around 8 grams per cooked cup (182 grams)
Other Nutrition Information: Low glycemic index, promoting stable blood sugar levels. Good source of manganese, magnesium, and iron.

Whole Wheat Pasta:
Recommended Daily Intake:
Men: 38 grams
Women: 25 grams
Adult: 25-38 grams
Young (12-18 years): 20-31 grams
Kids (4-8 years): 14 grams
Fiber Content: Approximately 6 grams per cooked cup (140 grams)
Other Nutrition Information: Contains fewer calories and more nutrients than refined pasta. Rich in B-vitamins, iron, and protein.

Whole Grain Bread:
Recommended Daily Intake:
Men: 38 grams
Women: 25 grams
Adult: 25-38 grams
Young (12-18 years): 20-31 grams
Kids (4-8 years): 14 grams
Fiber Content: Varies depending on the brand and type, typically 2-4 grams per slice (30-40 grams)
Other Nutrition Information: Contains complex carbohydrates, promoting sustained energy levels. Good source of folate, niacin, and zinc.

Buckwheat:
Recommended Daily Intake:
Men: 38 grams
Women: 25 grams
Adult: 25-38 grams
Young (12-18 years): 20-31 grams
Kids (4-8 years): 14 grams
Fiber Content: Roughly 5 grams per cooked cup (168 grams)
Other Nutrition Information: Gluten-free grain, rich in antioxidants like rutin. Contains essential amino acids and minerals such as manganese and magnesium.

Farro:
Recommended Daily Intake:
Men: 38 grams
Women: 25 grams
Adult: 25-38 grams
Young (12-18 years): 20-31 grams
Kids (4-8 years): 14 grams
Fiber Content: Approximately 8 grams per cooked cup (194 grams)
Other Nutrition Information: Rich in protein, promoting muscle health and repair. Contains vitamins B3, B5, and zinc.

Millet:
Recommended Daily Intake:
Men: 38 grams

Women: 25 grams
Adult: 25-38 grams
Young (12-18 years): 20-31 grams
Kids (4-8 years): 14 grams
Fiber Content: Around 2 grams per cooked cup (174 grams)
Other Nutrition Information: Gluten-free grain, rich in antioxidants like polyphenols. Contains magnesium, phosphorus, and B-vitamins.

The function of dietary fiber in the digestive system

Dietary fiber, also known as roughage or bulk, is the indigestible portion of plant foods that passes relatively intact through the digestive system. While it's not broken down or absorbed like other nutrients, such as carbohydrates, proteins, and fats, dietary fiber plays several important roles in the digestive system. Here's a detailed look at its functions:

Promotes Healthy Digestion: Fiber adds bulk to stool, which helps move it through the digestive tract more efficiently. This promotes regular bowel movements and prevents constipation. Insoluble fiber, in particular, acts like a sponge, absorbing water and softening stool, making it easier to pass.

Prevents Constipation: One of the primary functions of dietary fiber is to prevent and alleviate constipation. Insoluble fiber adds bulk to stool, while soluble fiber absorbs water, both of which help to soften and bulk up stool, making it easier to pass.

Supports Gut Health: Fiber acts as a prebiotic, providing fuel for beneficial gut bacteria in the colon. These bacteria ferment fiber, producing short-chain fatty acids (SCFAs) like acetate, propionate, and butyrate. SCFAs are important for maintaining a healthy gut environment, nourishing the cells lining the colon, and reducing inflammation.

Regulates Blood Sugar Levels: Soluble fiber slows down the absorption of sugar from the digestive tract into the bloodstream, helping to regulate blood sugar levels. By slowing the digestion and absorption of carbohydrates, fiber prevents spikes in blood sugar levels after meals, which is beneficial for individuals with diabetes or insulin resistance.

Lowers Cholesterol Levels: Soluble fiber binds to cholesterol in the digestive tract, preventing its absorption into the bloodstream. This helps lower LDL (bad) cholesterol levels, reducing the risk of heart disease and stroke. Foods rich in soluble fiber, such as oats, barley, beans, and legumes, are particularly effective at lowering cholesterol.

Promotes Weight Management: High fiber foods tend to be more filling and satisfying than low fiber foods. Fiber slows down digestion and promotes satiety, reducing hunger and calorie intake. By adding bulk to meals without adding excess calories, fiber helps support weight management and may aid in weight loss.

Prevents Diverticular Disease: Diverticula are small pouches that can form in the colon. When these pouches become inflamed or infected, it leads to diverticulitis. High fiber diets help prevent diverticular disease by keeping stool soft and preventing pressure buildup in the colon, reducing the risk of diverticula formation and inflammation.

Supports Healthy Weight: Fiber-rich foods often require more chewing, which slows down eating and allows for better regulation of hunger cues. Additionally, fiber adds bulk to the diet without adding excess calories, promoting a feeling of fullness and satisfaction with fewer calories consumed.

Promotes Regular Bowel Movements: Dietary fiber helps to regulate bowel movements by adding bulk to stool and promoting the movement of waste through the digestive tract. This can help prevent constipation and alleviate symptoms of irritable bowel syndrome (IBS).

Reduces the Risk of Colorectal Cancer: High fiber diets have been associated with a reduced risk of colorectal cancer. Fiber helps to keep the colon clean and healthy by promoting regular bowel movements and reducing inflammation. Additionally, the fermentation of fiber in the colon produces SCFAs, which may have anti-cancer effects.

Step-by-step tips on how to add more fiber to your diet

Incorporating more fiber into your diet is an excellent way to promote digestive health, regulate blood sugar levels, lower cholesterol, and maintain a healthy weight. Here are step-by-step tips on how to add more fiber to your diet:

Assess Your Current Intake: Begin by evaluating your current diet to determine how much fiber you're consuming on a daily basis. Keep a food journal or use a nutrition tracking app to record your meals and calculate your fiber intake. The recommended daily intake of fiber is 25 grams for women and 38 grams for men, but individual needs may vary.

Set Realistic Goals: Start by setting achievable goals for increasing your fiber intake. Gradually increasing fiber intake over time allows your digestive system to adjust and minimizes the risk of discomfort from gas, bloating, or abdominal cramps. Aim to add an extra 5 grams of fiber per day until you reach your target intake.

Choose High Fiber Foods: Incorporate a variety of high fiber foods into your meals and snacks. Focus on whole, minimally processed foods such as fruits, vegetables, whole grains, legumes, nuts, and seeds.

These foods are naturally rich in fiber, vitamins, minerals, and antioxidants.

Eat Whole Grains: Replace refined grains with whole grains to boost your fiber intake. Choose whole grain options such as brown rice, quinoa, barley, oats, whole wheat bread, whole grain pasta, and whole grain cereals. Look for products with "whole grain" or "whole wheat" listed as the first ingredient.

Load Up on Fruits and Vegetables: Make fruits and vegetables the stars of your meals by filling half of your plate with these fiber-rich foods. Aim for a variety of colorful options to ensure you get a wide range of nutrients. Incorporate fresh, frozen, or canned fruits and vegetables into your meals and snacks.

Snack on Fiber-Rich Foods: Choose high fiber snacks to keep you satisfied between meals. Snack on raw vegetables with hummus, fresh fruit with nut butter, Greek yogurt with berries, trail mix with nuts and seeds, or whole grain crackers with cheese.

Add Beans and Legumes: Incorporate beans, lentils, chickpeas, and other legumes into your meals to boost fiber content. Add beans to soups, stews, salads, stir-fries, tacos, and burritos. Experiment with different varieties of beans and legumes to keep your meals exciting.

Include Nuts and Seeds: Sprinkle nuts and seeds such as almonds, walnuts, chia seeds, and flaxseeds on top

　　　　

of salads, yogurt, oatmeal, or smoothie bowls. Add them to homemade granola, energy bars, or baked goods for extra fiber, protein, and healthy fats.
Read Food Labels: When grocery shopping, read food labels to identify high fiber options. Look for products that contain whole grains, fruits, vegetables, nuts, and seeds listed as the first few ingredients. Aim for foods with at least 3-5 grams of fiber per serving.

Stay Hydrated: Drink plenty of water throughout the day to help fiber move through your digestive system smoothly. Fiber absorbs water and swells in the digestive tract, so adequate hydration is essential for optimal digestion and bowel regularity.

Experiment with Recipes: Get creative in the kitchen by experimenting with new recipes that feature high fiber ingredients. Try adding vegetables to omelets, smoothies, and pasta dishes. Make hearty salads with a mix of leafy greens, beans, grains, and nuts. Explore different cooking methods such as roasting, steaming, sautéing, and grilling to enhance the flavor and texture of high fiber foods.

Be Mindful of Portions: While increasing your fiber intake is beneficial, it's essential to be mindful of portion sizes, especially if you're adding high fiber foods that are also calorie-dense. Balance your meals with a mix of fiber-rich foods, lean proteins, healthy fats, and complex carbohydrates to create balanced and satisfying meals.

Symptoms that you are eating too much fiber intake

While fiber is essential for digestive health and overall well-being, consuming too much fiber can lead to certain symptoms and discomfort for some individuals. Here are detailed symptoms that you may be eating too much fiber:

Bloating: Excessive fiber intake can lead to bloating, discomfort, and feelings of fullness due to the fermentation of fiber in the colon. This fermentation produces gases such as methane, hydrogen, and carbon dioxide, which can accumulate in the digestive tract and cause bloating.

Gas and Flatulence: Increased fiber intake can result in excessive gas production, leading to frequent passing of gas (flatulence). This is particularly common with certain types of fiber, such as insoluble fiber found in fruits, vegetables, and whole grains.

Abdominal Cramps: Consuming too much fiber can cause abdominal cramps or discomfort, especially in individuals with sensitive digestive systems. The expansion of fiber in the digestive tract can lead to irritation and spasms in the gastrointestinal muscles.

Diarrhea: While fiber is known for promoting regular bowel movements, consuming excessive amounts of fiber, especially insoluble fiber, can have a laxative effect and lead to diarrhea. This occurs because fiber absorbs water in the digestive tract, which can soften stool and increase bowel motility.

Constipation: Paradoxically, excessive fiber intake can also lead to constipation in some individuals. Insoluble fiber, in particular, can bulk up stool and promote regular bowel movements, but excessive intake without adequate hydration may result in hard, dry stools that are difficult to pass.

Nutrient Malabsorption: Consuming too much insoluble fiber can interfere with the absorption of certain minerals, such as calcium, iron, zinc, and magnesium. This occurs because insoluble fiber binds to minerals in the digestive tract, making them less available for absorption by the body.

Stomach Upset: Some individuals may experience stomach upset or gastrointestinal discomfort, including nausea or vomiting, with excessive fiber intake. This may be due to the rapid fermentation of fiber in the colon, leading to increased gas production and discomfort.

Feeling Too Full: Fiber-rich foods tend to be more filling and satiating, which can be beneficial for weight management. However, consuming too much fiber at once may leave you feeling overly full and uncomfortable, especially if you're not used to a high fiber diet.

Dehydration: Fiber absorbs water in the digestive tract, which can lead to dehydration if you're not drinking enough fluids. It's essential to drink plenty of water throughout the day, especially when increasing fiber intake, to prevent dehydration and promote optimal digestion.

Intestinal Blockage (Rare): In extreme cases of excessive fiber intake, particularly if combined with inadequate fluid intake, there is a risk of intestinal blockage or impaction. This is more common with soluble fiber supplements, such as psyllium husk, rather than naturally occurring dietary fiber.

If you experience any of these symptoms after increasing your fiber intake, it's essential to reassess your diet and make adjustments accordingly. Gradually increasing fiber intake over time, staying hydrated, and choosing a variety of fiber-rich foods can help prevent discomfort and promote optimal digestive health.

Breakfast

Overnight Oats with Berries and Almonds

Ingredients:
1/2 cup rolled oats
1/2 cup almond milk
1/4 cup Greek yogurt
1 tablespoon chia seeds
1/4 cup mixed berries (strawberries, blueberries, raspberries)
1 tablespoon sliced almonds
1 teaspoon honey or maple syrup (optional)

Preparation:
In a jar or bowl, combine rolled oats, almond milk, Greek yogurt, and chia seeds.
Stir well, cover, and refrigerate overnight.
In the morning, top with mixed berries, sliced almonds, and a drizzle of honey or maple syrup if desired.
Prep Time: 5 minutes (+overnight soaking)
Fiber Content: Approximately 8 grams per serving
Nutrition Information: Provides a good source of fiber, protein, healthy fats, vitamins, and minerals.

Avocado Toast with Poached Egg:

Ingredients:
2 slices whole grain bread
1 ripe avocado
2 eggs
Salt and pepper to taste
Optional toppings: cherry tomatoes, arugula, red pepper flakes

Preparation:
Toast the whole grain bread slices until golden brown.
Mash the ripe avocado and spread it evenly onto the toasted bread slices.
Poach the eggs until the whites are set but the yolks are still runny.
Place one poached egg on each avocado toast, season with salt and pepper, and add optional toppings if desired.
Prep Time: 10 minutes
Fiber Content: Approximately 7 grams per serving
Nutrition Information: Rich in fiber, healthy fats, protein, vitamins, and minerals.

Greek Yogurt Parfait with Granola and Fruit:

Ingredients:
1 cup Greek yogurt (plain or flavored)
1/4 cup granola (choose a high fiber variety)
1/2 cup mixed fresh fruit (such as sliced bananas, berries, or diced mango)
Optional toppings: honey, nuts, seeds

Preparation:
In a glass or bowl, layer Greek yogurt, granola, and mixed fresh fruit.
Repeat the layers until the ingredients are used up, ending with a layer of fruit on top.
Drizzle with honey and sprinkle with nuts or seeds if desired.
Prep Time: 5 minutes
Fiber Content: Approximately 6 grams per serving
Nutrition Information: Provides a good source of protein, calcium, fiber, vitamins, and antioxidants.

Spinach and Feta Egg Muffins:

Ingredients:
6 eggs
1 cup fresh spinach, chopped
1/4 cup crumbled feta cheese
Salt and pepper to taste
Optional add-ins: diced bell peppers, onions, mushrooms

Preparation:
Preheat the oven to 350°F (175°C) and grease a muffin tin.
In a bowl, beat the eggs and season with salt and pepper.
Stir in the chopped spinach, crumbled feta cheese, and any optional add-ins.
Pour the egg mixture evenly into the muffin cups, filling each about 3/4 full.
Bake for 20-25 minutes or until the egg muffins are set and lightly golden.
Allow to cool slightly before serving.
Prep Time: 10 minutes (+baking time)
Fiber Content: Approximately 2 grams per serving
Nutrition Information: High in protein, vitamins, minerals, and antioxidants, with moderate fiber content.

Whole Grain Pancakes with Berry Compote:

Ingredients:
1 cup whole wheat flour
1 tablespoon baking powder
1 tablespoon honey or maple syrup
1 cup almond milk
1 egg
1 teaspoon vanilla extract
1 cup mixed berries (fresh or frozen)
1 tablespoon water

Preparation:
In a bowl, whisk together the whole wheat flour, baking powder, honey or maple syrup, almond milk, egg, and vanilla extract until smooth.
Heat a non-stick skillet or griddle over medium heat and lightly grease with cooking spray or oil.
Pour 1/4 cup of the pancake batter onto the skillet and cook until bubbles form on the surface, then flip and cook until golden brown.
In a small saucepan, heat the mixed berries with water over medium heat until softened, stirring occasionally to make a compote.
Serve the pancakes topped with the berry compote.
Prep Time: 20 minutes
Fiber Content: Approximately 5 grams per serving
Nutrition Information: Provides a good source of fiber, whole grains, vitamins, and antioxidants

Lunch

Quinoa Salad with Chickpeas and Vegetables:

Ingredients:
1 cup cooked quinoa
1/2 cup cooked chickpeas (canned or cooked from dry)
1 cup mixed vegetables (such as diced cucumber, cherry tomatoes, bell peppers, and red onion)
2 tablespoons chopped fresh parsley

1 tablespoon olive oil
1 tablespoon lemon juice
Salt and pepper to taste

Preparation:
In a large bowl, combine cooked quinoa, chickpeas,
mixed vegetables, and chopped parsley.
Drizzle with olive oil and lemon juice, then season
with salt and pepper to taste.
Toss everything together until well combined.
Serve chilled or at room temperature.
Prep Time: 15 minutes
Fiber Content: Approximately 8 grams per serving
Nutrition Information: High in fiber, protein,
vitamins, minerals, and antioxidants.

Black Bean and Vegetable Quesadillas:

Ingredients:
4 whole grain tortillas
1 cup cooked black beans (canned or cooked from
dry)
1 cup mixed vegetables (such as bell peppers, onions,
corn, and spinach)
1/2 cup shredded cheese (such as cheddar or
Monterey Jack)
1/4 cup salsa
Cooking spray or olive oil for greasing

Preparation:
Heat a non-stick skillet over medium heat and lightly
grease with cooking spray or olive oil.

Place one tortilla in the skillet and top with half of the black beans, mixed vegetables, shredded cheese, and salsa.
Place another tortilla on top and press down gently.
Cook for 2-3 minutes on each side or until the tortilla is golden brown and the cheese is melted.
Repeat with the remaining ingredients to make another quesadilla.
Slice the quesadillas into wedges and serve hot.
Prep Time: 20 minutes
Fiber Content: Approximately 9 grams per serving
Nutrition Information: Provides a good source of fiber, protein, calcium, and vitamins.

Mediterranean Chickpea Salad:

Ingredients:
1 can (15 ounces) chickpeas, drained and rinsed
1 cup diced cucumber
1 cup cherry tomatoes, halved
1/4 cup diced red onion
1/4 cup chopped fresh parsley
2 tablespoons lemon juice
2 tablespoons extra virgin olive oil
1 teaspoon minced garlic
Salt and pepper to taste

Preparation:
In a large bowl, combine chickpeas, cucumber, cherry tomatoes, red onion, and parsley.

In a small bowl, whisk together lemon juice, olive oil, minced garlic, salt, and pepper to make the dressing.
Pour the dressing over the chickpea salad and toss until well coated.
Serve immediately or refrigerate for later.
Prep Time: 10 minutes
Fiber Content: Approximately 10 grams per serving
Nutrition Information: High in fiber, protein, vitamins, minerals, and healthy fats.

Vegetable Stir-Fry with Tofu:

Ingredients:
1 block (14 ounces) extra firm tofu, pressed and cubed
2 cups mixed vegetables (such as bell peppers, broccoli, carrots, snap peas, and mushrooms)
2 cloves garlic, minced
2 tablespoons low-sodium soy sauce
1 tablespoon sesame oil
1 tablespoon rice vinegar
1 teaspoon grated ginger
Cooked brown rice for serving

Preparation:
Heat sesame oil in a large skillet or wok over medium-high heat.
Add tofu cubes and cook until golden brown on all sides, then remove from the skillet and set aside.

In the same skillet, add mixed vegetables and minced garlic. Stir-fry for 3-4 minutes until vegetables are tender-crisp.

Return tofu to the skillet, then add soy sauce, rice vinegar, and grated ginger. Stir well to combine.

Cook for another 2-3 minutes until everything is heated through.

Serve the vegetable stir-fry with cooked brown rice.

Prep Time: 25 minutes

Fiber Content: Approximately 7 grams per serving

Nutrition Information: Provides a good source of fiber, protein, vitamins, and minerals.

Dinner

Chickpea and Vegetable Curry:

Ingredients:

1 can (15 ounces) chickpeas, drained and rinsed

1 cup diced tomatoes

1 cup chopped mixed vegetables (such as bell peppers, carrots, and peas)

1 onion, finely chopped

2 cloves garlic, minced

1 tablespoon curry powder

1 teaspoon ground turmeric

1 teaspoon ground cumin

1/2 teaspoon ground ginger

1 can (13.5 ounces) coconut milk

Salt and pepper to taste

Cooked brown rice or quinoa for serving

Preparation:
In a large skillet or saucepan, sauté the onion and garlic in olive oil until softened.
Add the diced tomatoes, mixed vegetables, chickpeas, and spices (curry powder, turmeric, cumin, and ginger). Stir well to combine.
Pour in the coconut milk and bring the mixture to a simmer.
Cook for 15-20 minutes, stirring occasionally, until the vegetables are tender and the flavors have melded together.
Season with salt and pepper to taste.
Serve the chickpea and vegetable curry over cooked brown rice or quinoa.
Prep Time: 30 minutes
Fiber Content: Approximately 10 grams per serving
Nutrition Information: Provides a good source of fiber, protein, vitamins, and minerals.

Grilled Salmon with Roasted Vegetables:

Ingredients:
4 salmon fillets
2 cups mixed vegetables (such as bell peppers, zucchini, carrots, and onions), cut into bite-sized pieces
2 tablespoons olive oil
1 teaspoon dried herbs (such as thyme, rosemary, or oregano)
Salt and pepper to taste

Preparation:
Preheat the grill to medium-high heat.
In a bowl, toss the mixed vegetables with olive oil, dried herbs, salt, and pepper until evenly coated.
Place the salmon fillets and seasoned vegetables on the grill.
Grill the salmon for 4-5 minutes per side, or until cooked through and flaky.
Grill the vegetables for 8-10 minutes, or until tender and slightly charred.
Serve the grilled salmon with roasted vegetables on the side.
Prep Time: 20 minutes
Fiber Content: Approximately 5 grams per serving
Nutrition Information: High in protein, omega-3 fatty acids, fiber, vitamins, and minerals.

Vegetable and Lentil Soup:

Ingredients:
1 cup dried lentils, rinsed and drained
4 cups vegetable broth
2 cups mixed vegetables (such as carrots, celery, onions, and spinach), diced
2 cloves garlic, minced
1 teaspoon dried thyme
1 teaspoon dried rosemary
Salt and pepper to taste
Fresh parsley for garnish

Preparation:
In a large pot, combine the dried lentils, vegetable broth, mixed vegetables, minced garlic, dried thyme, and dried rosemary.
Bring the mixture to a boil, then reduce the heat to low and simmer for 20-25 minutes, or until the lentils and vegetables are tender.
Season with salt and pepper to taste.
Ladle the vegetable and lentil soup into bowls and garnish with fresh parsley.
Prep Time: 30 minutes
Fiber Content: Approximately 12 grams per serving
Nutrition Information: Provides a good source of fiber, protein, vitamins, and minerals.

Stuffed Bell Peppers with Quinoa and Black Beans:

Ingredients:
4 large bell peppers, halved and seeds removed
1 cup cooked quinoa
1 cup cooked black beans (canned or cooked from dry)
1 cup diced tomatoes
1/2 cup diced onions
1/2 cup corn kernels (fresh or frozen)
1/2 cup shredded cheese (optional)
1 teaspoon chili powder

1/2 teaspoon ground cumin
Salt and pepper to taste

Preparation:
Preheat the oven to 375°F (190°C).
In a large bowl, mix together cooked quinoa, black beans, diced tomatoes, onions, corn kernels, chili powder, ground cumin, salt, and pepper.
Stuff each bell pepper half with the quinoa and black bean mixture.
Place the stuffed bell peppers in a baking dish, cover with foil, and bake for 30-35 minutes, or until the peppers are tender.
If desired, sprinkle shredded cheese over the stuffed peppers during the last 5 minutes of baking.
Serve the stuffed bell peppers hot.
Prep Time: 40 minutes
Fiber Content: Approximately 8 grams per serving

Desserts

Mixed Berry Chia Seed Pudding:

Ingredients:
1/4 cup chia seeds
1 cup almond milk (or any milk of choice)
1 tablespoon honey or maple syrup
1/2 teaspoon vanilla extract
1/2 cup mixed berries (such as strawberries, blueberries, raspberries)

Preparation:
In a bowl, mix chia seeds, almond milk, honey or maple syrup, and vanilla extract.
Stir well and let it sit for 10 minutes, then stir again to break up any clumps.
Cover and refrigerate for at least 2 hours or overnight until the mixture thickens and forms a pudding-like consistency.
Before serving, layer the chia pudding with mixed berries in a glass or bowl.
Optional: garnish with additional berries or a drizzle of honey.
Prep Time: 5 minutes (+chilling time)
Fiber Content: Approximately 10 grams per serving
Recommended Daily Intake: Men - 38 grams, Women - 25 grams, Kids - varies by age, but generally 19-25 grams

Baked Apple with Cinnamon and Almonds:

Ingredients:
2 apples (such as Granny Smith or Honeycrisp)
2 tablespoons chopped almonds
1 tablespoon honey or maple syrup
1/2 teaspoon ground cinnamon

Preparation:
Preheat the oven to 375°F (190°C).
Core the apples and cut them in half horizontally.

Place the apple halves, cut side up, on a baking sheet lined with parchment paper.
In a small bowl, mix chopped almonds, honey or maple syrup, and ground cinnamon.
Spoon the almond mixture into the center of each apple half.
Bake for 20-25 minutes or until the apples are tender and lightly golden.
Serve the baked apples warm, optionally with a dollop of Greek yogurt or a sprinkle of additional cinnamon.
Prep Time: 10 minutes
Fiber Content: Approximately 6 grams per serving

Chocolate Avocado Mousse:

Ingredients:
2 ripe avocados
1/4 cup cocoa powder
1/4 cup honey or maple syrup
1 teaspoon vanilla extract
Pinch of salt
Optional toppings: sliced strawberries, shaved dark chocolate

Preparation:
Scoop the flesh of the avocados into a blender or food processor.
Add cocoa powder, honey or maple syrup, vanilla extract, and a pinch of salt.
Blend until smooth and creamy, scraping down the sides as needed.

Divide the chocolate avocado mousse into serving cups or bowls.

Chill in the refrigerator for at least 30 minutes before serving.

Garnish with sliced strawberries or shaved dark chocolate if desired.

Prep Time: 10 minutes (+chilling time)

Fiber Content: Approximately 7 grams per serving

Fruit and Yogurt Parfait:

Ingredients:

1 cup Greek yogurt (plain or flavored)

1/4 cup granola (choose a high fiber variety)

1/2 cup mixed fresh fruit (such as sliced bananas, berries, or diced mango)

Optional toppings: honey, nuts, seeds

Preparation:

In a glass or bowl, layer Greek yogurt, granola, and mixed fresh fruit.

Repeat the layers until the ingredients are used up, ending with a layer of fruit on top.

Drizzle with honey and sprinkle with nuts or seeds if desired.

Prep Time: 5 minutes

Fiber Content: Approximately 5 grams per serving

Snacks

Apple Slices with Peanut Butter:

Ingredients:
1 apple, sliced
2 tablespoons peanut butter (or almond butter)

Preparation:
Slice the apple into wedges or rounds.
Spread peanut butter on each apple slice.
Prep Time: 5 minutes
Fiber Content: Approximately 4 grams per serving
Recommended Daily Intake: Men - 38 grams, Women - 25 grams, Kids (ages 4-8) - 25 grams, Kids (ages 9-13) - 31 grams

Carrot Sticks with Hummus:

Ingredients:
2 carrots, peeled and cut into sticks
1/4 cup hummus

Preparation:
Peel and cut the carrots into stick shapes.
Serve the carrot sticks with hummus for dipping.
Prep Time: 5 minutes
Fiber Content: Approximately 3 grams per serving
Recommended Daily Intake: Refer to previous answer for daily fiber recommendations.

Trail Mix:

Ingredients:
1/4 cup almonds
1/4 cup walnuts
1/4 cup pumpkin seeds
1/4 cup dried cranberries
1/4 cup dark chocolate chips (optional)

Preparation:
Mix all the ingredients in a bowl.
Portion the trail mix into individual snack bags.
Prep Time: 5 minutes
Fiber Content: Approximately 5 grams per serving
Recommended Daily Intake: Refer to previous answer for daily fiber recommendations.

Greek Yogurt with Berries and Granola:

Ingredients:
1/2 cup Greek yogurt (plain or flavored)
1/4 cup mixed berries (such as strawberries, blueberries, raspberries)
2 tablespoons granola (choose a high-fiber variety)

Preparation:
In a bowl, layer Greek yogurt, mixed berries, and granola.
Repeat the layers if desired.
Prep Time: 5 minutes
Fiber Content: Approximately 3 grams per serving

Recommended Daily Intake: Refer to previous answer for daily fiber recommendations.

Edamame Beans:

Ingredients:
1 cup edamame beans (frozen or fresh)
Salt to taste

Preparation:
If using frozen edamame beans, thaw them by running them under warm water.
Bring a pot of water to a boil and add the edamame beans.
Cook for 3-5 minutes until tender, then drain.
Sprinkle it with salt to taste and serve warm or chilled.
Prep Time: 10 minutes
Fiber Content: Approximately 5 grams per serving
Recommended Daily Intake: Refer to previous answer for daily fiber recommendations.

Smoothies

Green Power Smoothie:

Ingredients:
1 cup spinach
1/2 cup kale
1/2 banana
1/2 cup pineapple chunks
1/2 cup Greek yogurt
1 tablespoon chia seeds
1 cup almond milk (or any milk of choice)

Preparation:
Add all ingredients to a blender.
Blend until smooth and creamy.
Add more almond milk if needed to reach desired consistency.
Prep Time: 5 minutes
Fiber Content: Approximately 7 grams per serving
Recommended Daily Intake: Men - 38 grams, Women - 25 grams, Kids (ages 4-8) - 25 grams, Kids (ages 9-13) - 31 grams

Berry Blast Smoothie:

Ingredients:
1/2 cup mixed berries (such as strawberries, blueberries, raspberries)
1/2 banana
1/4 cup rolled oats

1 tablespoon flaxseeds
1/2 cup Greek yogurt
1/2 cup almond milk (or any milk of choice)

Preparation:
Combine all ingredients in a blender.
Blend until smooth.
Add more almond milk if necessary to reach desired consistency.
Prep Time: 5 minutes
Fiber Content: Approximately 6 grams per serving

Tropical Paradise Smoothie:

Ingredients:
1/2 cup frozen mango chunks
1/2 cup frozen pineapple chunks
1/2 banana
1/2 cup spinach
1 tablespoon shredded coconut
1 tablespoon hemp seeds
1 cup coconut water (or any liquid of choice)

Preparation:
Place all ingredients in a blender.
Blend until smooth and creamy.
Add more coconut water if needed to adjust consistency.
Prep Time: 5 minutes
Fiber Content: Approximately 6 grams per serving

Peanut Butter Banana Smoothie:

Ingredients:
1 ripe banana
2 tablespoons peanut butter
1/4 cup rolled oats
1 tablespoon chia seeds
1 cup almond milk (or any milk of choice)
Optional: 1 tablespoon honey or maple syrup for sweetness

Preparation:
Combine all ingredients in a blender.
Blend until smooth.
Taste and add honey or maple syrup if desired for sweetness.
Prep Time: 5 minutes
Fiber Content: Approximately 8 grams per serving

Chocolate Avocado Smoothie:

Ingredients:
1 ripe avocado
1 tablespoon cocoa powder
1 tablespoon honey or maple syrup
1/2 cup Greek yogurt
1 cup almond milk (or any milk of choice)
Handful of ice cubes

Preparation:

Scoop the avocado flesh into a blender.

Add cocoa powder, honey or maple syrup, Greek yogurt, almond milk, and ice cubes.

Blend until smooth and creamy.

Prep Time: 5 minutes

Fiber Content: Approximately 7 grams per serving

BONUS: Comprehensive Shopping list

Fruits:
1. Apples
2. Bananas
3. Oranges
4. Berries (strawberries, blueberries, raspberries)
5. Pears
6. Kiwi
7. Mango
8. Avocado
9. Guava
10. Prunes

Vegetables:
1. Spinach
2. Kale
3. Broccoli
4. Brussels sprouts
5. Carrots

6. Bell peppers (red, green, yellow)
7. Cauliflower
8. Sweet potatoes
9. Artichokes
10. Peas (green peas, snap peas)

Legumes:
1. Lentils
2. Chickpeas
3. Black beans
4. Kidney beans
5. Pinto beans
6. Navy beans
7. Split peas
8. Lima beans
9. Edamame
10. Soybeans

Whole Grains:
1. Quinoa
2. Brown rice
3. Whole wheat bread
4. Oats (rolled oats, steel-cut oats)
5. Barley
6. Bulgur
7. Whole grain pasta
8. Farro
9. Millet
10. Buckwheat

Nuts and Seeds:
1. Almonds
2. Walnuts

3. Pistachios
4. Chia seeds
5. Flaxseeds
6. Pumpkin seeds
7. Sunflower seeds
8. Hemp seeds
9. Sesame seeds
10. Poppy seeds

Dairy and Alternatives:
1. Greek yogurt
2. Cottage cheese
3. Almond milk
4. Soy milk
5. Oat milk
6. Coconut milk (unsweetened)
7. Cashew cheese
8. Tofu
9. Tempeh
10. Kefir

Other Protein Sources:
1. Chicken breast
2. Turkey breast
3. Salmon
4. Tuna
5. Eggs
6. Lean beef
7. Pork loin
8. Shrimp
9. Cod
10. Seitan

Herbs and Spices:
1. Cinnamon
2. Turmeric
3. Ginger
4. Garlic
5. Basil
6. Oregano
7. Thyme
8. Rosemary
9. Cumin
10. Paprika

Healthy Fats:
1. Olive oil
2. Avocado oil
3. Coconut oil
4. Flaxseed oil
5. Almond butter
6. Peanut butter
7. Coconut butter
8. Tahini
9. Chia oil
10. Hemp oil

Condiments and Sauces:
1. Salsa (no added sugar)
2. Hummus
3. Mustard
4. Soy sauce (low sodium)
5. Balsamic vinegar

6. Apple cider vinegar
7. Hot sauce (without added sugar)
8. Tahini dressing
9. Guacamole
10. Pesto (with olive oil)

Beverages:
1. Green tea
2. Herbal teas
3. Sparkling water (plain or flavored)
4. Kombucha (low sugar)
5. Vegetable juice (low sodium)
6. Fruit-infused water
7. Almond milk (unsweetened)
8. Coconut water
9. Flavored water (without added sugar)
10. Protein shakes (low sugar)

Frozen Foods:
1. Frozen mixed berries
2. Frozen spinach
3. Frozen broccoli
4. Frozen peas
5. Frozen mango chunks
6. Frozen cauliflower rice
7. Frozen edamame
8. Frozen cherries
9. Frozen kale
10. Frozen mixed vegetables

Snacks:
1. Whole grain crackers
2. Rice cakes (whole grain)

3. Air-popped popcorn
4. Mixed nuts
5. Roasted chickpeas
6. Veggie chips
7. Granola bars (high fiber)
8. Rice cakes (whole grain)
9. Dark chocolate (70% cocoa or higher)
10. Trail mix (unsweetened)

Canned Goods:
1. Canned beans (no added salt)
2. Canned tomatoes
3. Canned pumpkin
4. Canned tuna (in water)
5. Canned salmon
6. Canned coconut milk (unsweetened)
7. Canned chickpeas (no added salt)
8. Canned lentils (no added salt)
9. Canned artichoke hearts
10. Canned green beans (no added salt)

Miscellaneous:
1. Nutritional yeast
2. Coconut flour
3. Whole grain tortillas
4. Brown rice cakes
5. Hemp protein powder
6. Flaxseed meal
7. Whole grain pita bread
8. Unsweetened applesauce
9. Miso paste
10. Dried fruit (unsweetened)

Specialty Foods:
1. Seaweed snacks
2. Spirulina powder
3. Wheat germ
4. Psyllium husk
5. Amaranth
6. Teff
7. Konjac noodles
8. Black rice
9. Farro
10. Soba noodles

Baking Supplies:
1. Whole wheat flour
2. Rolled oats
3. Baking powder
4. Baking soda
5. Almond flour
6. Coconut sugar
7. Agave nectar
8. Maple syrup
9. Raw honey
10. Unsweetened cocoa powder

Conclusion

In conclusion, incorporating high fiber foods into your diet is a simple yet powerful way to promote overall health and well-being. From fruits and vegetables to whole grains, legumes, nuts, and seeds, there's a wide variety of delicious and nutrient-rich options available to help you meet your daily fiber needs.

By including high fiber foods in your meals and snacks, you can support digestive health, maintain a healthy weight, and reduce the risk of chronic diseases such as heart disease, diabetes, and certain types of cancer. Fiber-rich foods not only provide essential nutrients but also contribute to feelings of fullness and satiety, helping you manage hunger and maintain energy levels throughout the day.

Whether you're aiming to increase your fiber intake for better digestive health or to achieve other health goals, remember to choose a diverse range of high fiber foods and incorporate them into your diet gradually. Additionally, make sure to stay hydrated and listen to your body's signals to ensure a balanced and sustainable approach to nutrition.

Incorporating high fiber foods into your daily meals and snacks is not only beneficial for your health but also adds variety, flavor, and enjoyment to your diet.

With the knowledge gained from this high fiber food list, you can make informed choices to create delicious and nutritious meals that support your overall well-being for years to come

I trust this culinary journey has not only ignited your passion for wholesome eating but has also become a haven of inspiration, solace, and invaluable insights. Each carefully curated recipe within this High fiber food list reflects a dedication to excellence, with a profound understanding of the comprehensive guide to the high fiber diet.

Crafted with meticulous attention to detail, these recipes go beyond the realm of mere sustenance; they are a testament to the art of nourishing the body and soul.

Your reviews, experiences, and insights are needed to guide me on improving this book.

Every evaluation is a stepping stone for refinement, as I aspire to tailor this food list to surpass your expectations. Let's engage in a dialogue that transcends the pages, creating a connection that resonates with your culinary preferences and well-being goals.

Warm Culinary Regards,

Tina Feldman

www.ingramcontent.com/pod-product-compliance
Lightning Source LLC
Chambersburg PA
CBHW051656250726
48653CB00007B/2699